PORK EATING

THE GREAT RISK TO HUMAN HEALTH

NEW REVISED EXPANDED EDITION 2019

ABOLADE NKOSI TAYO

PORK EATING

THE GREAT RISK TO HUMAN HEALTH
NEW REVISED EXPANDED EDITION 2019
Abolade Nkosi Tayo

Disclaimer:

Wherever a vegetable or any food is recommended as having medicinal properties, this is not intended as medical advice. You should consult your doctor or physician for advice on any particular disease you may be diagnosed with. This is only to be understood as information, and no cure is recommended for any specific diseases. Consult your Doctor/ Physician or Healthcare provider for all medical advice.

TABLE OF CONTENTS

FOREWORD

It is with great concern that I wrote this book, I feel it necessary, even though there are a few books addressing the dangers of pork consumption as food. Some books did not go deep enough to reveal that even cows, goats, chickens, sheep etc.. were being fed the remains of dead, diseased pigs by way of the feed they were ingesting. So even though someone might boast. "I eat beef, mutton, chicken and goat, but I do not touch the filthy hog", in reality they were still eating hog, as the same animals they ate were eating pork products in their feed.

This is very wrong, as the cow, the goat and the sheep are all vegetarians and they were being fed not only the remains of dead diseased pigs (hogs), but also chickens, cows etc.These animals were forced to deviate from their norm (vegetarianism) and partake of animals like themselves and in addition pork was included in the formula of the feed.

Who knows what metabolic, psychological and genetic damages were-done to these vegetarian animals.Who is to say that the germs from the pork did not infect the cows, causing mad cow disease, who is to say for sure that it cannot alter any of the systems in these animals?

Who is to say that the prevalence of crime, violence and other unaccepted behavior cannot be traced to the consumption of meat from cows, goats, sheep and chickens tainted with the pork laced feed fed to these animals.

Look at the situation with cancer, caused by wrong diets, smoking - even cigarettes haven't escaped, having in addition its myriad of cancer causing properties, the cigarettes are treated with pork (read Chapter 5 of this book) products. Are some people so stubborn as to ignore these facts. I know a man who is so arrogant about smoking that he gets mad when you to show him the dangers of smoking, what example is he setting for his children, how much love does he really have for them, to subject them to second hand and side hand smoke, does he really care? I doubt it as cigarette smoking is a waste of money, wasting your health, time, and besides being self destructive, it also destroys other people's health and lives, how selfish can a cigarette smoker be.

The fact of the matter is, pork is so well spread out, that if you are not careful you may be using it in some form, soaps, toiletries, medicine and some processed foods etc..

Do you think the producers of pork really care about anyone's health, the main reason, the number one goal is to make money, and pork makes money. Despite the fact that the religious books of the Jews (Torah), the Christians (The Bible) and the Muslims (The Holy Qur'an) condemn the use of pork as food, and these books are very old, the Creator in His wisdom did not permit mankind to eat the Hog If you look at Genesis in the Bible you would see that mankind originally had vegetarian nutrition, it is only after the flood, when all vegetation was destroyed, that man was permitted to eat animals and only the clean ones at that.

A. If Noah had eaten one hog, there would not be any today, as the Bible clearly states two of the unclean to preserve seed, but seven of the clean, so anyone who wants to insinuate that after the flood Noah could have eaten any or all of the animals you are wrong, only the clean ones were his choice.

Then there is the question of pets, how safe is it to have pets in the home, read Chapter 9, you would be shocked.

All in all, this book addresses the problems which most of the pork books have left out, at the end of this book there is a list of books I recommend that you read, as they are all good, they contain valuable information for mankind's wellbeing, I hope you enjoy reading my book, and encourage others to do so, thank you.

(A)That is what Genesis 6:19, 20 say, but Genesis 7:2,3 say something else.

I only made that reference as some Christians may be reading this book.

Genesis 6:19, 20 say 2 of every kind (clean and unclean) Genesis 7:2,3 say 7 each of the clean, and 2 each of the unclean. My other books take up that issue, this one only deals with the connection of pigs' meat in relation to your health.

CHAPTER 1

WHAT IS FOOD?

Food is safe nutrients ingested into the digestive system, providing building blocks, and other essential necessary for human nutrition and well being.

I must point out here to the die-hard (dying from the numerous diseases caused by eating the pig as food), that I know they will say that pork has proteins etc.., but I must make a few points, centipedes, scorpions etc.., their flesh contain proteins and other nutrients, that doesn't make them fit as food for humans. There are poisonous plants, and they all contain vitamins, minerals and proteins but that still doesn't make them fit for human consumption. The criterion should not be, what can be used as food in them, but what about the poisons, the germs, the disease causing bacteria.

Containing all (these) minuses, pork would definitely have to be ruled out as food, as it would not be safe as food. The very make up of the pig rules it out as food, it is a scavenger (read Chapter 3), it is disease and germ ridden (read Chapter 2), the Bible condemns it as food, the Holy Qur'an also condemns the eating of the pig as food (read Chapter 6).

Food is not just anything you put into your mouth. Did you ever stop to think why there are so many headache concoctions, so many concoctions for indigestion, constipation etc..

There is a vicious cycle, the present food choices contribute to these ailments, so naturally, you eat a junk diet, you get constipated you have to blast (yes blast) an exit for the filth, whereas if you ate the right foods you would never suffer from constipation. I am never constipated and I never take any of those constipation blasters.

Food should be nutritious, you can snack on a mango, a banana and not have to worry about constipation and some headaches caused by constipation. It takes less time to snack on something nutritious, and safe than some fries or other junk food or junk drink.

Have patience, you take so much care of your car, your external appearance (nice clothing etc.), then what about the more important you, your health, do you really care?

If so, begin today to change the norm and start enjoying good healthy, nutritious food.

CHAPTER 2

A LOOK AT THE DISEASE CAUSING GERMS CARRIED BY THE PIG

"Trichinosis causes fever, muscle aches and swelling around the eyes" (1)

Why should anyone want to subject themselves to not only discomfort, but disease and sickness, and some instances death.

"In the January 1942 issue of Life and Health, there is a statement estimating that our present hog crop may provide us with 60, 000, 000 trichinae-infested meals. (2)

That was in 1942, but the danger is even greater in this present time, even more infested, disease causing meals.

"Brucellosis or swine abortion … in the hog, brucellosis causes abortion and sterility, the disease is difficult to diagnose and practically impossible to cure". (3)

Brucellosis in humans can lead to disease infecting the productive organs, which can lead to sterility and abortion, also other problems in the body.

"Hot dogs are a potential source of a type of organism causing sporotrichinosis, a skin disease characterized by a string of nodules developing upward along the path of the lymphatic". (4)

Sporotrichinosis affects humans internally and externally and the damages are really extensive.

> "Paragonimus lives in the lungs of pigs. It was discovered by Dr. Mason in 1880. It is a common parasite which causes pneumonia in pigs. There is still no way of killing the parasites in the tissues, neither has anyone found a method of expelling them" (5)

Look at that frightening situation, regarding the question of what "Paragonimus" does to pigs, and you ingesting that meat, which will bring those parasites into your body.

Then the big problem will be getting rid of them, and who knows what health problems known and unknown that they will cause.

> "Hook worm -any of certain blood sucking nematode worms equipped with mouth hooks, which feed off of the lining of the intestines of men and animals, often causing a disease characterized by severe anemia." (6)

Hook worms are spread to man by the consumption of pork.

As a child I ate pork, and I can tell you from personal experience, that I had very unpleasant situations with hookworms.

My mother gave us worm expelling medicine which she made, and there in our feces, you could see the worms. Now the dangers of having those worms in your body are that when you feel sick, the doctor may overlook or do not see the worm problem and misdiagnose you for another problem, not even related to what is going on inside of you, think about that, as it can lead to other health problems.

> "Round worm - a nematode, esp. Ascaries Lambricoides a parasite infesting the intestines of vertebrates." (7).

Roundworms are transmitted from the hog to mankind, through the consumption of its flesh and also coming in contact with its meat in the slaughterhouse etc.

"Roundworms, these are from four to ten inches long, pointed at the ends like earthworms, but of a yellow - white color or tinged with red. They naturally inhabit the upper parts of the bowels, but wander about and are often vomited from the stomach.

"They may thus be found in the nose or throat. They are ordinarily seen in the excrement, and a white, mucous discharge from the bowels is occasionally mistaken for them." (8)

Plus there are many other worms, germs and diseases carried by the hog and transmitted to humans through their consumption of the hog and its products.

Look at this disturbing and sickening health situation, is it really worth risking your health, by eating hog (pig, swine) look at the length of these worms.

This is why so many people eat so much, as the worms are consuming much of the food they are eating, also making them sick, as they are not only found in the upper parts of the bowels, but move around inside your body, this can be avoided, it's up to you.

"The common tapeworms are of two varieties; beef and pork tapeworms, caused by eating of the raw or imperfectly cooked meats ... There is a great danger to children with tapeworms conveying some of the eggs from the parts about the rectum to their mouths, through sucking their fingers. In this event the immature tapeworms enter the body and attack other organs, thus endangering the life of the patient". (9)

Remember what I said earlier, in the foreword of this book, on what is being fed to cows etc, and they are becoming infected, just like pigs are.

Just pause for a moment and take a look at the serious effects of the tapeworms in the human body, also the great danger to children. Remember that the tape worms attack other organs in the body, endangering life.

What is the obsession in eating anything which will cause harm to you in so many ways.

> "Roundworms, these parasites of men are identical with those found in pigs, they belong to the same species. It means that the worm which is found in pork is quite easily transferred to human-beings where it does a lot of damage." (10)

Roundworms are transferred from pork to human beings, where they can infest the body, causing health issues eventually

> "The human incidence of human infection with the pork Tapeworm varies throughout the world. In his now classic Report, "This Wormy World, (1947) Stoll estimated that 2.5 million persons throughout the world were infected with the organism." (11)

In 1947 that was the situation, you can just imagine presently, what that number will be, with so much more pork being made available nationwide and worldwide.

> "The ordinary tapeworm is from twenty to fifty feet long, made up of white, flattened joints or segments. The head is the size of a pinhead, and the neck is not much thicker than a thread, but the middle and lower part of the body is from a quarter to half an inch wide. The presence of the worm is recognized by the escape of pieces of it in the excrement every few days" (12)

Look at the size of an ordinary tapeworm, and slowly but surely it is going to undermine the health of whichever body it inhabits.

"Tapeworms are much less common in this country since meat has been under closer scrutiny at the time of slaughter, as most cases arise from infested pigs or cattle who contain the worm in their guts ...Most symptoms arise from the colicky pains and loss or appetite that the tapeworm causes." (13)

Even the quality of cow's meat presently is being jeopardized by what happens in some of the places where these animals are reared.

Read my other books "DISTURBING CONSEQUENCES" AND "SCIENCE GONE MAD" for more information on this subject.

But do not let "much less common" make you feel too secure, as it doesn't mean that it does not exist. And there are so many other health risks in eating pork, that it should be avoided.

Tapeworm - any of the various flat or tapelike cestode worms, as those belonging to the genus Taemia, parasitic when adult in the alimentary canal of man and other vertebrates, and usually characterized by having the larval and adult stages in different hosts." (14)

The bottom line is that "Tapeworms" are not "friends", neither do they contribute to good health or well-being.

"Both the pigs and the chicken on a farm showed Campylobacter, a germ capable of causing diarrhea. The origin of a boy's diarrhea was definitely diagnosed when his own stools showed the same Campylobacter". (15)

Does it make any sense to consume as food, an animal (the hog) so infested with germs, diseases ,worms and who knows what else, and all these ailments are easily transmitted to humans. Is there a scarcity of food so that mankind must sink so low to eat sickness, germs and diseases, wake up.

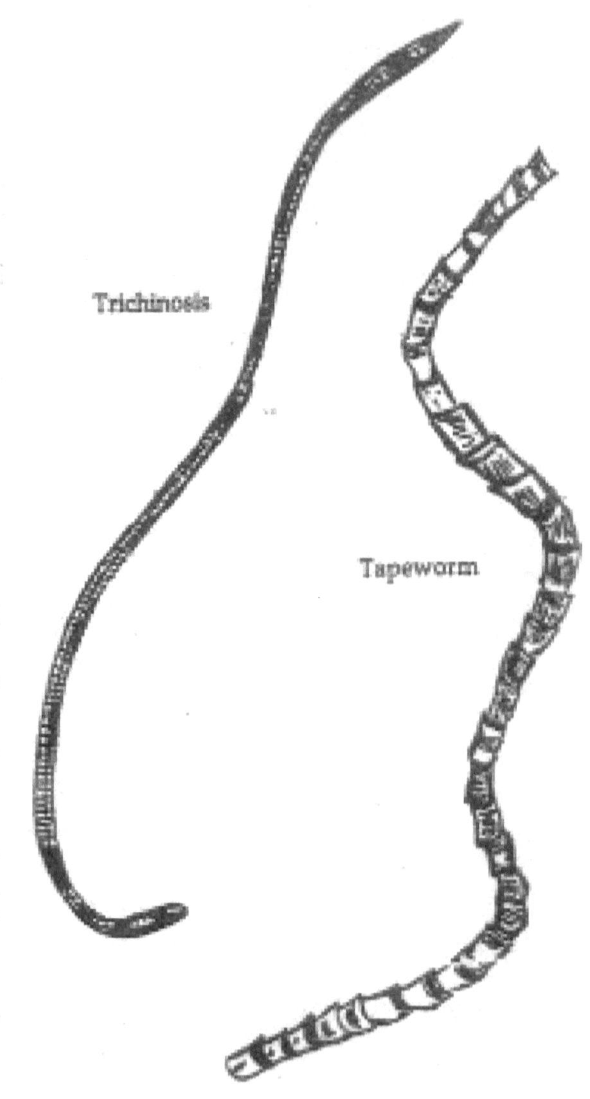
Trichinoeis
Tapeworm

References

1. The Animal Connection by Agatha Thrash MD and Calvin Thrash MD page 7

2. The Hog - Should It Be Used For Food? by C. Leonard Vories page 16

3. What The Holy Qur'an, Bible and Medical Say About Pork By Din Rana page 15

4. The Animal Connection by Agatha Thrash MD and Calvin Thrash MD page 7

5. What The Holy Qur'an, Bible and Medical Say About Pork By Din Rana pages 12, 13

6. The Living Webster Encyclopedic Dictionary of the English Language 1975 Edition page 462

7. The Living Webster Encyclopedia Dictionary of the English Language 1975 Edition page 837

8. World Scope Family Library - The Family Physician by Dr. Herman Pomeranz and Dr. Irvis S. Koll page 295

9. World Scope Family Library - The Family Physician by Dr. Herman Pomeranz and Dr. Irvis S. Koll page 296

10. What The Holy Qur'an, Bible and Medical Say About Pork By Din Rana page 11

11. What The Holy Qur'an, Bible and Medical Say About Pork By Din Rana page 11

12. World Scope Family Library - The Family Physician by Dr. Herman Pomeranz and Dr. Irvis S. Koll page 296

13. Understanding Disease – A Health Practitioner's Handbook by John Ball page 46

14. The Living Webster Encyclopedic Dictionary of the English Language 1975 Edition page 1004

15. The Animal Connection by Agatha Trash MD and Calvin Thrash MD page 6

CHAPTER 3

THE PIG, A SCAVENGER IN THE ANIMAL KINGDOM

The pig is the perfect scavenger on the land, as it is an eating machine, eating literally anything that it can get its teeth into, the scavenger par excellence in the animal kingdom.

"Farmers know that when they are feeding cattle it will also pay them to keep hogs, so that the hogs can follow after the cattle, eat the filth from the cattle, and thus turn it into pork for the public market."(1)

The pigs were actually used for two purposes, to clean up the mess, and then to be sold as pork.

Many thousands of hens and hundreds of hogs were kept on this farm. When hens would die, they would be put into burlap sacks. After some had lain in the sacks for days and the odor from them had become unbearable, they were then loaded onto a truck and hauled to the hog pen where they became feed for the hogs. This procedure was not unusual on this farm. It was the regular way of disposing of the dead hens", (2)

In Trinidad in the Caribbean, the hogs are fed something called hog food. When I was a child, people who owned hogs would leave buckets at friends, and they would throw in all the skins and sour food (stale food), as in those days few persons owned refrigerators, so the life of food cooked on any day was short, it had to be eaten within a certain time frame, so any of this food left over would be thrown in this bucket and covered.

The persons rearing hogs would not come every day, as he (or she) had several buckets at various friends, so when your turn comes: he would pick up the bucket with stale, sour, smelly food and dump all into a big pot and make hog food, then he (or she) would feed this grimy, smelly food to the hogs who literally licked it all up, and got fatter and fatter and fatter.

"It is illegal to feed raw garbage to hogs. However, processed (cooked) garbage is legal.

> This cooked garbage is so-called animal food causes anemia, ulcers and systematic disorders (disease in the entire pig), antibiotics such as copper sulphate (a poison) is fed to the hogs to increase their growth. It also causes nerve and brain damage, senility and decreases the lifespan. Of course, these chemicals are passed along to the consumer of animal flesh. (3)

The whole problem is that no animals in their natural habitat, eat anything cooked. And another problem is that most of the raw garbage were already cooked, therefore, in the first instance, all of the garbage were already devitalized, and cooking it a second time, even made it worse.

So the pigs were actually being fed twice dead food, therefore it made the pigs sick.And in addition, the poisons fed to them to increase their growth, make them even more dangerous to be consumed as food.

"Carnivore and saprophytes which batter on the offal of terrestrial life - the domesticated pig eating its own excreta, the domesticated chicken eating human and animal excreta, all of them eating dead and decaying flesh - are content with poor food supplies. The appetites of scavengers grow with what they feed upon, so that they tend to eat more and more filth." (4)

This is so abnoxious, how can these creatures be considered healthy to eat?

"We know that God had some purpose in creating the hog and we may well believe that He designed that it should be a scavenger in the animal kingdom, for we cannot think of one beast among all the beasts of nature which could better serve as a scavenger than the hog.Everyone who knows anything about the hog knows that it is, by nature, a dirty creature. All have heard the trite old expression, "As dirty as a hog," when people wanted to make a comparison to something filthy. See the brute as he wallows in the mud." (5)

This is a true story, in Trinidad, in the Caribbean, I taught Martial Arts all over the island, I remembered once I was in a town called Point Fortin which is situated in the southern part of the island.It was December and lots of households boiled hams, fried bacon, etc.. In the household I was in, I noted they never cooked any pork or pork products, I asked the lady of the house, "Why?". She replied that she has a son who is a seaman, and when he returned from one of his sailings, he told her this, "Mamie, when I visited Colombia, I saw a pig (swine) eating a dead dog, please whenever you cook ham or any pork products, I don't want any." Needless to say, his mother never cooked any of that filthy meat again, and I visited them on several occasions and never saw any pork products cooked in that house.

As a child I would run away from home without my mother's permission and go to the dump (La Basse) in Port of Spain, Trinidad, and something that caught my eyes, was a huge pig (there were others also) with piglets, they lived at the dump and they enjoyed living there, where they had all the filth they could ingest everyday. You could have heard their gleeful grunts as they ate and ate, those garbage piles containing old food. and rotting flesh, filth (human and animal) and the hogs were just happy, the biggest hogs l have ever seen, were in that dump, called "La Basse" in Trinidad.

Without a doubt the structure of the hog, the very built-in outlet in its foot where pus runs out, attest to the fact, that it was created to dispose of garbage, and it really does a splendid job in doing so.

Do you think that of all the animals eaten by mankind, the filthiest, the scavenger par-excellence is the most used as food, in medicine, to make several items and as an additive in myriad's of food and other products, it is almost as if they are putting this dirty, filthy beast on a high pinnacle and exalting it as "GOOD FOOD", what a tragedy, why all this madness?

References

1. The Hog ~ Should It Be Used For Food? - by C Leonard Vories page 10

2. The Hog - Should It Be Used For Food? - by C Leonard Vories page 12

3. African Holistic Health by Llaila O Afrika page 129

4. Superior Nutrition by H.M. Shelton pages 68, 69

5. The Hog - Should It Be Used For Food? - by C Leonard Vories page 10

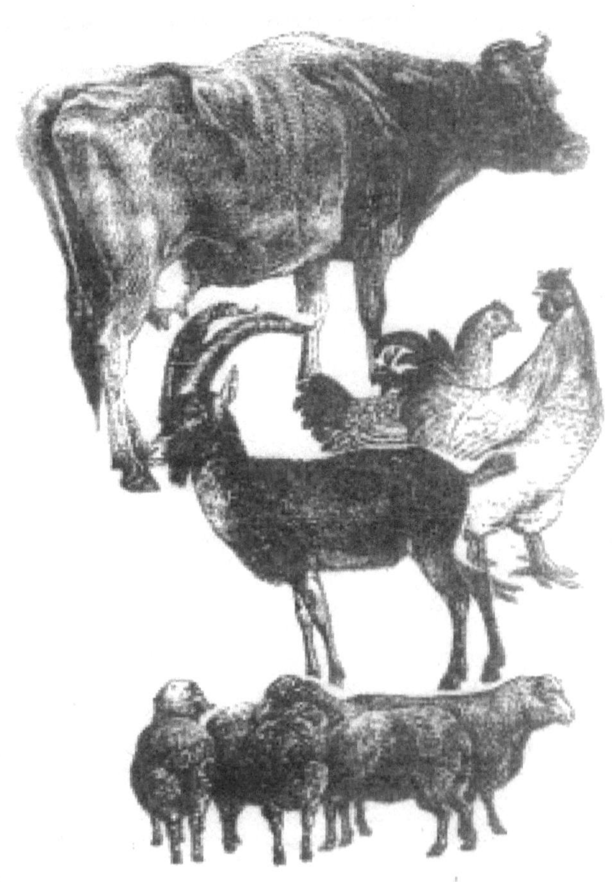

CHAPTER 4

THE MAIN REASONS FOR THE REARING OF PIGS (HOGS, SWINE)

"Farmers know that when they are feeding cattle it will also pay them to keep hogs so that the hogs can follow after the cattle, eat the filth from the cattle, and thus turn it into pork for the public market." (1)

A few years ago on many farms that was the norm, but it is still done in a more sophisticated, so-called scientific way as you will see, keep on reading.

"The pig still functioned as the garbage disposal during early American times, what they ate was generally called "slop" which contained scraps of food, trash, human and animal refuse, rotten vegetables and the like. They got rid of it quickly, saved the farmer money by not requiring special feed, and remained on spot for the next bucket of "slop" to be dumped in their sty" (2)

Not only was this practice time saving, but also very economical to the farmers.

"Many thousands of hens and hundreds of hogs were kept on this farm. When hens would die, they would be put into burlap sacks. After some has lain in the sacks for days and the odor from them had become unbearable, they were then; loaded onto a truck and hauled to the hog pen where they became feed for the hogs. This procedure was not unusual on this farm. It was the regular way of disposing of the hens." (3)

As I said before the system has become more sophisticated, where all sorts of dead animals, chicken and other animals waste are processed into an animal feed, more later on.

"Cancerous hogs and diseased hogs are masked by giving them inoculations. Moreover, pork has never been graded. Consequently, the ratio of fat to meat is solely controlled by the meat industry, not the federal government. Fat is the storage place for high concentrations of poisonous chemicals." (4)

Some Muslims who advocate eating swine (pig, hog) fat should take note that the fat is the storehouse for the poisonous chemicals – beware! I am not crazy,there are some Muslims who say it is ok to eat the pig,I heard it from them ,personally,so I am relating it to you,first hand.

"One radio pitch man who is very vigorous in his denunciation of vegetarianism and in his insistence that man must eat animal foods, gives away hams over the radio as a means of inducing people to listen to his meat-selling talks. It is well, always, when one of these men begin his task for flesh-eating, to stop him long enough to ask what he is selling and who is paying his salary, If you know what he is selling and who is paying his salary, you may then know what he "thinks and why he says what he does". "Money talks." It also writes, as Sinclair has Shown." (5)

Yes even in this present 21st century some proponents of "you must eat animal products to be healthy," still belting out that propaganda, using all the media.

Yet still millions of people are giving up that habit and enjoying better health. A long, long time ago when animals were reared naturally and humanely, the dangers were lessened, but now it is just astronomical.

"Americans have an appetite for vegetarian animals...... Before these vegetarians end up on a plate, they are fattened with protein supplements, a meat and bone meal made from the remains of slaughtered or diseased chickens, cows, pigs and other livestock .... Feeding animal parts to plant-eaters is a perversion of nature for Scott Williams, executive director of the Farm Animal Reform Movement, a national group that wants to end human consumption of livestock." (6)

This is the point I have been hinting to, earlier in this chapter, a combination of all those remains, sometimes combined with feathers, chicken excrement etc. rendered into a feed for the animals.Is this ethical, right or healthy for the animals and in extension humans who will be eating their flesh?

"We've asked all cattle producers, beef and diary, to cease feeding ruminant derived proteins to keep American cows free of mad cow disease, said Gary Weber director of animal health for the National Cattlemen's Beef Association, which represents 230, 000 cattlemen... The ban "would cripple us," said Ben Heirnann, President of De Kalb Feeds Inc. in Rock Falls, Illinois. "I don't know how we could cope with the economic loss if we couldn't use it."Feed companies and renders companies that grind up animal remains for protein supplements argue there is no scientific proof that mad cow disease is caused by feeding ruminant based proteins to ruminant animals." (7)

The insane part of all the reasons given for rearing pigs is the end motive, making money, regardless of how much evidence is piled up against human ingesting the pig (hog).No amount of evidence can convince the producers, no evidence from The Bible, The Holy Qur'an, Medical Science and personal experiences could change their attitudes.

The reasons they give, the pig is a good garbage disposal unit on a chicken or cow farm, it serves a dual purpose, it cleans up the mess and the cost of rearing the pig is minimal.

They will say that the practice of using the pig as a garbage disposal, is a thing of the past, but wait, it has become more scientific (?) and more subtle, as not only the pigs are fed this new garbage, but chickens, cows, sheep etc.

Then you have persons who are paid and sponsored by these pork producers, so naturally they have to protect their interest at all costs. Then look at the outbreak of mad cow disease in England, the feed fed to vegetarian animals - cows, goats, sheep etc., is laced with the remains of the hogs, this doesn't need a scientist to give a scientific reason; common sense can tell you that hogs are the carriers of so many diseases and germs. On top of that, you are feeding that filth to vegetarian animals, what scientific findings can state without a doubt, that this kind of feeding would not affect the health of animals involved, who knows?

And the health of those who eat the animals ingesting that type of despicable feed, are at risk, as can be seen by those who contracted and died from mad cow disease.

It is interesting to note here that it was reported that one vegetarian also died from mad-cow disease.

It was also stated that he was on a vegetarian diet for about two years. This just goes to show how deadly mad-cow disease is, as he may have been infected two or more years earlier.

References

1. The Hog - Should It Be Used For Food? by C. Leonard Vories page 12

2. How Not To Eat Pork by Shahrazad Ali page 21

3. The Hog - Should It Be Used For Food? by C. Leonard Vories page 12

4. African Holistic Health by Llaila O Afrika page 129

5. Superior Nutrition by H. M. Shelton page 73

6. Chicago Sun-Times Thursday July 1996 page 13 Inset

7. Chicago Sun-Times Thursday July 25 1996 page 12

CHAPTER 5

SOME PRODUCTS CONTAINING PORK

Some people are careful in avoiding pork and its by products, but they still smoke cigarettes, well I have some bad news for you.

"Also note that tobacco manufacturers treat cigarettes tobacco leaves with chemical pork derivatives substance to maintain its freshness" (1)

SOAP

Read the labels carefully, any time you see tallow or tallowate, leave it alone as the tallow could be from the pig's fat.In any event you should avoid any soap with all those chemical additions, look for natural soap without additives, soap made from coconut, olive etc.Some supermarkets carry a few, but sometimes you have to look very carefully.

The health Food stores carry a wider range, also vendors at Flea Markets, yard sales, special Events, who are into health and well being carry them sometimes.

TOOTHPASTE

Same thing goes for toothpaste, avoid all the long chemical additives, there are herbal toothpastes without those chemical additives, some supermarkets carry them, the Health Food Stores have a wider range. Good toothpaste without any pork or other animals derivatives can be found, if you make that extra effort to locate them.

MISCELLANEOUS FOOD ITEMS

Try your very best to eat and drink naturally, as it is very wise to avoid all processed foods with all those additives, "natural" on the label may not be what you think.By avoiding all processed foods, you won't have to worry about what's in them.

Try your best to use fresh produce every day, avoid all processed oils, as with the benefits there are risks. You can get coconut oil from eating coconut or making your own coconut milk at home. Same thing goes for many of the other oils, eat an olive, sunflower seeds, flax seeds, hemp seeds etc.

Avoid canola oil and don't even think of eating what canola oil is made from. A word of caution some peanut butters contain lard, make your own at home it's easy.

COSMETICS

A whole bunch of cosmetics contain animal derivatives and some include the pig, go natural, the Health Food Stores have a whole bunch of natural healthy products.

FISH

Even some processed fish products contain questionable ingredients, just leave them alone.

"Look for lard, animal shortening, shortening, gelatin, calcium, emulsifiers, stabilizers and protein" (2)

Another thing to look for, whenever a label says animal fat, this is not good enough, as you must ask yourself this question, "which animal?".

"In an effort to salvage inedible tallow (product from the swine) and grease, the USDA is developing methods of adding them to livestock feed". (3)

As I said earlier, the best move is to avoid all processed foods with all those questionable additives, as they contribute to a lot of diseases, which you can avoid, by eating natural.

References

1. Halal Watch – Article "Smoking is Un-Islamic" page 11

2. How Not to Eat Pork by Shaharazad Ali Page 38

3. Consumer Beware! By Beatrice Trump page 113

CHAPTER 6

WHAT SOME RELIGIONS SAY ABOUT PIG CONSUMPTION AS FOOD – CHRISTIANS (SEVENTH DAY ADVENTISTS), JEWS (JUDAISM), MUSLIMS (ISLAM)

Since the Christians and the Jews accept the Old Testament as their holy book, the quotations I will make, would be the position of the Christians(Seventh Day Adventists etc.) and the Jews (Judaism).

GENESIS 7:1 - 3 (KIV)

1. And the Lord said unto Noah, Come thou and thy house into the ark; for thee have I seen righteous before me in this generation.

2. *Of every clean beast thou shalt take thee by sevens,* the male and his female: and of the beasts that are not clean by two, the male and his female.

3. Of fowls of the air by sevens, the male and the female; to keep the seed alive upon the face of all the earth

GENESIS 9:3

> 3. *Every moving thing that liveth shall be meat for you*; even as the green herb have I given you all things

LEVITICUS 11:7; (KJV)

> 7. And the swine, though he divide the hoof, and be cloven-footed, yet he cheweth not the cud; he is unclean to you.

DEUTERONOMY 14:8; (KJV)

> 8. And the swine because it divideth the hoof, yet cheweth not the cud, it is unclean unto you: ye shall not eat of their flesh, nor touch their dead carcass.

ISAIAH 65:4; (KJV)

> 4. Which remain among the graves, and lodge in the monuments; *which eat swine's flesh*, and broth of abominable things is in their vessels;

ISAIAH 66:17; (KJV)

> 17. They that sanctity themselves, and purify themselves in the gardens behind one tree in the midst, eating swine's flesh, and the abomination, and the mouse, shall be consumed together, saith the Lord.

I will now quote from the New Testament, the holy book accepted by the Christians (Seventh Day Adventists and other Christians.)

ACTS 10:12 -14; (KJV)

> 12. Wherein were all manner of four footed beasts of the earth, and wild beasts, and creeping things, and fowls of the air.

> 13. And there came a voice to him, Rise, Peter; kill and eat.

14. But Peter said, Not so, Lord; *for I have never eaten anything that is common or unclean.*

This was a vision Acts 10:12-14: which Peter had, it was not in reference to food as you would see from the verses that followed, but the point I want to make is that Peter although he was a Christian he still followed the law of clean and unclean animals, this does not change the Levitical admonitions, this is not a license to eat the swine.

I now quote from the Holy Qur'an, the Final Revelation from Allah to mankind, the Holy Book wherein is guidance for all mankind (Muslims and non-Muslims)

Holy Quran 5:3;

3. Forbidden to you (for food) are: dead meat, blood, the flesh of swine

Holy Quran 2:173;

173. He hath only forbidden you dead meat, and blood and the flesh of swine,

Holy Quran 6:145;

145. Say: I find not in the Message received by me by any (meat) forbidden to be eaten by one who wishes to eat it, unless it be dead meat, or blood poured forth, or that flesh of swine

The reason for my adding the following material to my book, is that having dialog with some Muslims, it was brought to my attention, that their understanding of Sura 6:146 is that the swine was not unlawful to the Jews.

And furthermore, in conjunction with Sura 5:5,... The food of the people of the book is lawful for you (Muslims), this makes the swine lawful.I was really amazed at that statement, and what made me even more amazed was the there were other Muslims sharing that belief.

But does the Qur'an support that understanding?

Before we take a closer look at Sura 6:146, let us look at a few verses on the same topic.

Sura 5:3-5,

3. Forbidden you is carrion and blood, and the flesh of the swine, and whatever has been killed in the name of some other than God (Allah), and whatever has been strangled, or killed by a blow or a fall, or by goring, or that which has been mauled by wild beast unless slaughtered while still alive, and that which has been slaughtered at altars is forbidden, and also dividing the meat by casting lots with arrows. All this is sinful. Today the unbelievers have lost every hope of (despoiling) your creed; so do not fear them, fear me. Today I have perfected your system of belief and bestowed my favours upon you in full, and have chosen submission (al-islam) as the creed for you. If one of you is driven by hunger (to eat the forbidden) without the evil intent of sinning, then God (Allah) is forgiving and kind.

4. They ask you what is lawful for them; Say: "All things are lawful for you that are clean, and what the trained hunting animals take for you as you have trained them in the light of God's (Allah's) teachings, but read over them the names of God (Allah), and fear (straying from the path of) God (Allah) is swift in the reckoning".

5. On this day all things that are clean have been made lawful for you; and made lawful for you is the food of the people of the Book, as your food is made lawful for them…

Sura 2:168, 169, 172, 173

168. O men, eat only the things of the earth that are lawful and good.

Do not walk in the footsteps of Satan, your acknowledged enemy.

169. He will ask you to indulge in evil, indecency, and to speak lies of God (Allah) you cannot even conceive.

172. O believers, eat what is good of the food we have given you, and be grateful to God (Allah), if indeed you are obedient to Him.

173. Forbidden to you are carrion and blood, and the flesh of the swine, and that which has been consecrated (or killed) in the name of any other than God (Allah).

If one is obliged by necessity to eat it without intending to transgress, or reverting to it, he is not guilty of sin; for God (Allah) is forgiving and kind.

Sura 6:119

119. And why should you not eat of what over which the name of God (Allah) has been pronounced, when He has made it distinctly clear what is forbidden, unless you are constrained to do so.

Surely many (men) mislead others into following their vain desires through lack of knowledge. Your Lord certainly knows the transgressors. Refer also to Sura 6:118, Sura 6:121.

Sura 6:141, 142, 145

141. It is He who grew the gardens, trellised and bowered, and palm trees and land sown with corn and many other seeds, and olives and pomegranates, alike. So eat of their fruits when they are in fruit and give on the day of harvesting His due, and do not be extravagant.

142. He has created beasts of burden and cattle for slaughter. So eat of what God (Allah) has given you for food, and do not walk in the footsteps of Satan who is surely your declared enemy.

143. You tell them "In all the commands revealed to me I find nothing which men are forbidden to eat except carrion and running blood and flesh of swine for it is unclean, or meat consecrated in the name of some other than God (Allah), which is profane.

But if one is constrained to eat of those without craving or reverting to it, then surely, your Lord is forgiving and kind.

Sura 16:114, 115, 116, 118

114. Eat the good and lawful things that God (Allah) has given you, and be grateful for the bounty of God (Allah), if you really worship Him.

115. He has forbidden carrion and blood and the flesh of swine, and what has been killed in the name of any other but God (Allah); but if one is driven by necessity (to eat it) without craving or reverting to it, then God (Allah) is forgiving and kind.

116. Do not utter the lies your tongues make up;

"This is lawful, and this is forbidden," in order to impute lies to God (Allah); for they who impute lies to God (Allah) will not find fulfillment.

118. We have already told you what we have forbidden the Jews. We did not wrong them, they wronged themselves.

Surah 23:51.

51. O ye apostles, eat things that are clean, and do things that are good. We are surely cognisant of what you do.

Sura 5:100

> 100. Tell them: "The unclean and the pure are not equal, even though the abundance of the unclean may be pleasing to you". So fear God (Allah), O men of wisdom; you may haply find success.

So it is evident where food is mentioned where Allah says to eat, that they are clean, good and lawful.

Examples are Sura 35:3. The food mentioned here would be clean, good and lawful, other verses are Sura 34:15, 24, Allah is consistent in what He says, so there is no need to go over what is clean, good and lawful whenever food is mentioned by Allah, as He already has stated so many times, what is good, clean and lawful.

Allah specifically speaks of clean and unclean, go back to Sura 6:145, Sura 5:4, Sura 23:51, Sura 5:100.

Now let us get back to Sura 6:146, but this time let us read from verse 145 which is the context * to verse 146

Sura 6:145, 146,

> 145. You tell them: "In all the commands revealed to me I find nothing which men have been forbidden to eat except carrion and running blood and flesh of the swine for it is unclean, or meat consecrated in the name of some other than God (Allah), which is profane.
>
> 146. 146. We made unlawful for the Jews all animals with claws or nails, and the fat of the oxen and sheep, except that on their backs or their instestines, or which remains attached to their bones.

I must make a short note here, in the word for word translation of Sura 6:145, "eater" is there instead of "men", which makes it even better.

As the verse is applicable to all who are eating, so the prohibition is to all who are eating, which includes everyone, Jews, Christians, Muslims, everyone, "all".

But let us take a closer look at Sura 6: 146, it begins with "And" (wa) in the word for word translation, and many translations begin with "And".

So my understanding of that verse 146, is that the Jews fell under 145, and 146 has additional restrictions for the Jews as a punishment.

*** Context**

1. Parts that surrounds or clarity a word or passage.

2. relevant circumstances page 125. The Oxford Desk Dictionary .

Other verses to consider are Sura 16:115, 116, 117, 118 especially verse 118 in conjunction with verse 115, I will make the point at the end of this chapter.

Sura 6:145, 146 cover what they were forbidden not just verse 146.

Another verse they like to parade to support their view is Sura 3:93,

93. To the children of Israel was lawful all food * except what Israel forbade himself before the Torah was revealed.

* Food here does not include all species and is in perfect harmony with Sura 6: 145, as even in the Bible, before Israel came into existence, there were clean and unclean animals, go to Genesis 7:8, Genesis 9:3 does not contradict Genesis 7:8, as Noah already knew what was clean and what was unclean, so every moving thing that liveth had a clear meaning for him.

So what Israel forbade for himself, was excluded some of what was lawful, but they (Israel) made it on their own forbidden, so even here, there is no room for assuming that the swine was permissible for the Jews at any time.

So it is abundantly clear that the swine (the living garbage disposal unit) was unfit for food, it is in the Jewish, Christian scriptures, and The Holy

Qur'an :it is not fit for food, it was never permitted as food, even when all vegetation was destroyed by the flood, only the clean animals were permitted to be eaten.

I must make a point here, the Bible clearly states that originally, before the flood mankind's diet was vegetarian.

GENESIS 1:29; (KJV)

> 29. And God said, Behold, I have given you every herb bearing Seed, which is upon the face of all the earth, and every tree, in which is the fruit of a tree yielding seed; to you it shall be for meat.

After all vegetation was destroyed, this is when mankind was permitted to eat meat (the clean animals), but after vegetation began to grow again, man was not limited to eating clean animals, but his choice of vegetables, fruits ,grains etc.

Here is Biblical evidence that after the flood, a Vegetarian Diet, kept people healthy, let us turn to the book of Daniel.

DANIEL 1:10 - 16;

> 10. And the prince of the eunuchs said unto Daniel, I fear my lord the king, who hath appointed your meat and your drink. For why should he see your faces worse looking than the children which are of your sort? Then shall ye make me endanger my head to the king.

> 11. Then said Daniel to Melzar, whom the prince of the eunuchs had set over Daniel, Hananiah, Mishael, and Azariah.

> 12. Prove thy servants, I beseech thee, ten days; and let them give us pulse to eat, and water to drink.

13. Then let our countenance be looked upon before thee and the countenance of the children that eat of the portion of the king's meat: and as thou seest. Deal with thy servants.

14. So he consented to them in this matter, and proved them ten days.

15. And at the end of the ten days their countenance appeared fairer and fatter in flesh than all the children which did eat the portion of the king's meat.

16. Thus Melzar took away the portion of <u>their meat, and the wine</u> that they should drink; and gave them pulse.

Leviticus 11: 1 – 47, Leviticus 17:10, 12 – 14, Deuteronomy 14:3 – 21.

And in the Apocryphal books of 2nd and 4th Maccabees, the same message is there, 2 Maccabbees 6:18 – 23, 4 Maccabbees 5:1 – 27, 4 Maccabbees 6:1 – 30.

The whole understanding is why would there be so many verses in the Qur'an explicitly stating that the swine was unlawful for food, and then with a wrong understanding of one verse, the swine suddenly becomes lawful for food.

The Qur'an has no contradictions, so I do not see any in Sura 6:145, 146 and Sura 5:5.

As I close let us look at Sura 16:115 – 118, but particularly 115 and 118

Sura 16:115, 118, (Syed Vickar Ahamed Translation)

115. He has only forbidden for you, meat from dead (animals), and blood, and the flesh of swine, and any (food) over which the name of (anyone) other than Allah has been called upon. But if one is forced by (extreme) need, without willful disobedience, and not exceeding the rightful limits – Then, Allah is oft Forgiving, most merciful.

118. And for the Jews (also), we prohibited such things like what we have told you before: we did not do them any wrong, but they were used to doing wrong to themselves.

So there we have it ,read the in-between verses 116, 117, and it is clear that Sura 6:145 explains all that were forbidden to mankind, the Jews included and 146 were additional restrictions for the Jews as a punishment for them, so it is entirely wrong to assume that the swine was permissible for the Jews and in extension (food of the people of the Book) lawful to Muslims.

Sura 16:115 makes it clear what is forbidden and verse 118 makes it clear that it included the Jews.

So do not be misled by anyone teaching that the swine is permissible as food for Jews, Muslims or anyone, may Allah continue to guide us on His Right Path.

I take studying the Qur'an very seriously and I must say that I have seen no where in the Qur'an where any command is given to eat swine, except in situations where you do not have a choice, and even so when eating it, you are not to assume it as lawful.

Note # 1.

Recently, having dialog with some Muslims, it was stated more than once, that all species were permissible as food, that is incorrect for the following reasons.

a. There are poisonous plants which were not intended as food, and are highly toxic, Allah who knows everything would not recommend eating any of them.

b. There are marine species which are poisonous and toxic.

c. There are animals, which are poisonous and toxic

d. There are birds which are scavengers and are not fit as food for humans.

Note # 2: The swine is unclean

Allah has repeated many times about the prohibition of swine as food for humans, He has stated that the flesh of the swine is unclean – please read again Sura 6:145,

Note # 3: The Swine is forbidden as food for humans.

Read Sura 6:145, Sura 5:3, Sura 2:173, Sura 16:115.

Note # 4: Allah has made it clear that we are to eat things good, lawful, clean pure

Read Sura 5:4, Sura 2:168, 172, Sura 16:114, Sura 23:51, Sura 5:100.

Note # 5: In this present age some of the permissible foods have been tampered with and are not good.

Allah warned us about this in Sura 4:119.

> 119. And mislead them and tempt them, and order them to slit the ears of animals and <u>order them to alter God's (Allah's) creation"</u>.

He who holds Satan as friend in place of God will assuredly be damned to perdition.

In this present age, "Genetic Engineering is doing just that, altering Allah's creation". The so-called Scientists are placing genes from fish, animals etc., in plants, also altering fish, animals and a whole bunch of other madness.

Cloning animals and even messing with humans and the great increase in diseases and damage to human health and the environment is so visible.

Allah told us to eat what is clean, pure, good and lawful. Can a tomato or any fruits or vegetables be pure, good, clean and lawful, which have been engineered with animal and human genes?

There are pigs (swine) which have human DNA and other species engineered in them, are they good, clean, pure or lawful?

So Allah who never makes a mistake or short on words, has warned us against these Satanic deviations – affecting our food and environment.

And let me make you aware of what to avoid, you will notice

PLU # (numbers) on produce, they mean more than you can imagine

PLU # 9 with four numbers following example PLU # 93062 are organically grown.

PLU # 8 with four numbers following example PLU 82361 are Genetically modified.

PLU # 4 or 3 with three numbers following are conventional grown (non-gmo) or just 4 numbers.

So please read your labels to safeguard your health.

Note # 6 Prohibition of fat, except for a little that is hard to remove.

The toxins in animals are stored in the fat, also pesticides in the feed they eat, also the many chemicals factory reared animals, chickens, turkey etc.

The fat is literally a storehouse for all these poisons.

Presently all these poisons contributes to many major health problems, such as arthritis, stiffening of the joints, degeneration of many life supporting organs in the body,hardening of the arteries etc.

Note # 7. Allah specifically speaks of clean and unclean

Read Sura 6:145, Sura 5:4, Sura 23:51, Sura 5:100

So definitely as the clean are permissible, there are unclean and the swine is one of them – Sura 6:145. Look at Sura 5:4 only the clean are lawful, and even the hunting animals were trained in the light of Allah's teachings.

If you read Sura 34:15, 24 you will know from reading other verses which I referenced that _food_ would mean _clean_ and _good_, Allah has given each of us brains which we must use to think, to reflect, and to understand.

I must say with respect to the word of Allah- The Qur'an, I have clearly seen that all foods were not permissible, only the clean, pure, good and lawful ones.

And as one who has submitted to Allah, I must follow His clear guidance as shown in the Qur'an, and all over, the swine is forbidden as food, I have not seen one verse which says that the swine is clean, not forbidden and is good for Muslims or anyone to eat, except when there are no other choices.

So it is very obvious here that there were CLEAN AND UNCLEAN FOODS and ALLAH DOES NOT CONTRADICT HIMSELF, NEITHER DOES HE FORGET.

So whenever food is mentioned it must be remembered that what was and still is permissible are the clean foods, Sura 36:72, 73, Sura 36:33-36.

The Holy Quran states that Allah has provided food in abundance.

Holy Quran 55:10 - 13;

10. It is He who has spread out the earth for (His) creatures.

11. Therein is fruit and date palms producing spathes (enclosing dates):

12. Also corn, with (its) leaves and stalk for fodder, and sweet-smelling plants,

13. Then which of the favors of your Sustainer will you deny?

So the question is not about meat, it is about sustenance, do you think the permission to eat meat after the flood gave mankind the authority to drug, ill treat, manipulate, experiment and do all kinds of things to animals just so that they can be slaughtered?

Think about it, since there is an abundance of grains, beans, peas, vegetables, fruits. juices and myriad of foods, which does not entail suffering (for the sake of production) the animals etc., don't you think it is time that mankind stop and think, as all their arguments in favor of animal   protein superiority over vegetable protein has been debunked?

What about vegetarian scientists who have shown them over and over, the benefits of a vegetarian diet, they show you that the very reasoning of the "meat producers", can be used against them, if the vegetarian animals are best for food, then why not consume a vegetarian diet instead of eating the animal who eats a vegetarian diet, where is the wisdom?

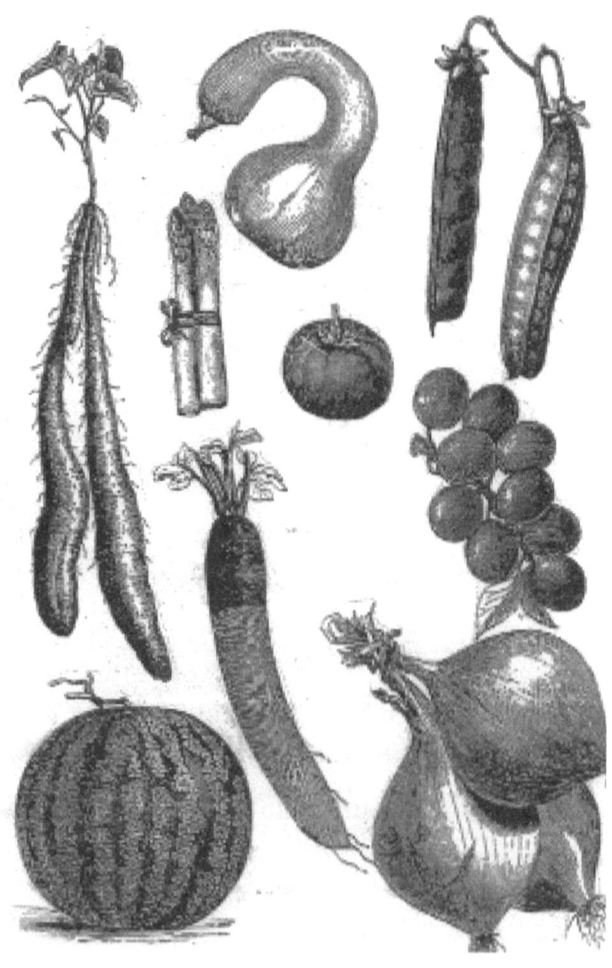

CHAPTER 7

IS IT WORTH THE RISK TO EAT PORK?

Seeing that the pig (swine) is so filthy, so germ ridden, so dangerous as food, why do people still insist on eating such filth?

Food does not necessitate your consuming garbage (pork) there is such a wide range to choose from, is the risk worth it? Read Chapter 1 again, What is food?

What about the myriad of germs, parasites, diseases etc. carried by the pig (hog, swine) Chapter 2 gives you a detailed look, read it again.

The pig (hog, swine) stands out as the animal with the most diseases, germs, parasites that are eaten by humans, are there no better choices? How can you be healthy by ingesting filth?

When you read the real reasons behind pig rearing, you might have second thoughts of consuming pork, read Chapter 4 again, you cannot afford to support big business at the expense of your health can you?

You have to be very careful about the items you use, bags soaps, cookies, candies, ice cream, foods etc, as there is this constant danger of you using products from the filthy pig, be careful, chapter 5 contains some hints.

Even among people who eat meat, there are a lot of them who shun pork, there are commandments against eating pork in the Jewish Scriptures, the Christian Scriptures and the Holy Qur'an.

All these scriptures were written a long time ago, when all this disease, parasite ,germ discoveries about the pig were not known to man, but the Holy Scriptures forbade the eating of the pig, this guidance came from the ALL-KNOWING CREATOR.

In many countries of the world, the pig is kept to dispose of garbage, it thrives on garbage, the fattest, biggest pigs can be found in the garbage dumps in a lot of small countries, and in the farms of bigger countries, to eat up the filth and dead chickens etc.

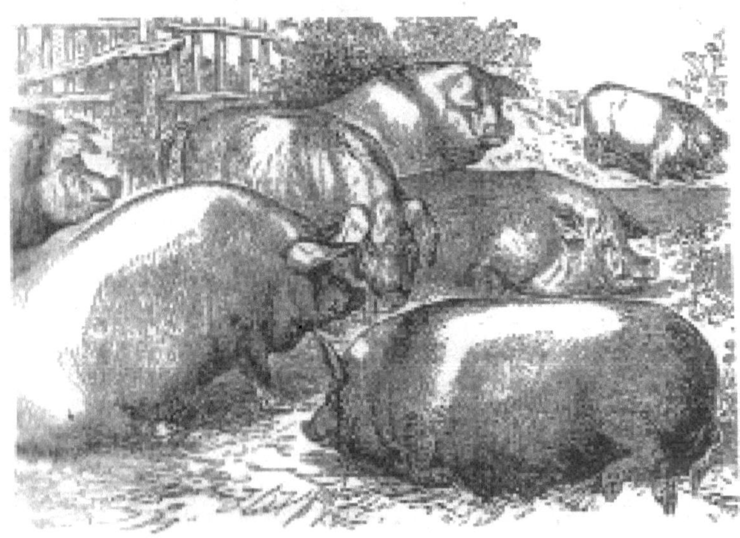

CHAPTER 8

THE DANGERS FACED IN CONSUMING ANY ANIMAL PRODUCTS, IN THIS MODERN AGE

As a result of the devious practices in meat production the question arises, "Is there any safe animal product, that's really fit for human consumption?"

I am sure you have read or heard or seen on television the outbreak of "mad cow disease", in England, I will now quote from an article I read in the Chicago Sun Times, Thursday July 25 edition titled "Mad Cow Disease: America's Response," page 12.

The article stated that, "failure to stop mad cow disease from entering the United States could endanger the public health and set off a panic that might damage the economy.

But there is no known way to stop this killer – just steps that might guard against it."

Quoting from a sub article titled "Animals part of livestock diet".

"Americans have an appetite for vegetarian animals.....Before those vegetarians end up on a plate, they are fattened with protein supplements, a meat and bone meal made from the remains of slaughtered diseased chickens, cows, pigs and other livestock."It's not a new practice", said Gary Weber, a director of animal health and meat inspection for the National Cattleman's Beef Association.""There's a belief of recycling these nutrient," he said, "For well over a hundred years, these protein by products have been part of an animal's diet ... (1)

Do those so-called Scientists ever think of adverse consequences, before they put their mad science into practice? How could they possible think that it would be good to feed vegetarian animals any animal by products, do they not think that this will have a negative reaction two ways, in the first instance to the animal and next to people who eat their tainted flesh?

"The animal diseases present a special medical and economic challenge. They include, several of the most widespread and serious infections of man. The experience of the past forty years lead us to assume that animal diseases will contribute even more to the burden of human disease in the future."(2)

Presently with all the advances in medical science, we have so many diseases, all types of cancers ,diabetes, arthritis etc, and what is frightening is that children are being diagnosed with diseases, which a long time ago only adults had.And a lot of the diseases from animal are taking a toll on human life.

"Tapeworms are much less common in this country since meat has been under closer scrutiny at the time of slaughter, as most cases arise from infested pigs or cattle who contain the worm in their gut."(3)

Tapeworms are still causing health problems in humans, even up to today.

"The United Nation's Food Agricultural Organization concluded that in the meat industry, diseases are more serious today than ever before. No current method of U.S. meat (includes seafood and poultry) inspection can assure non-contaminated and disease-free meat." (4)

Factory farms are responsible for this situation, due to overcrowding of the animals, also bad hygienic conditions, the use of so many chemicals.

Then, not every animal killed and sold as food is inspected.

> "There are other things that your immune system has to guard against, parasites that range in size from the tiny protozoa that squeeze into red blood cells and cause malaria, to the tapeworm that enters the body via uncooked fish and can grow up to (ugh!) thirty feet in length." (5)

That is so disturbing, imagine a worm in your body, up to thirty feet long, it most definitely will be consuming some of the food you eat. This in turn would be jeopardizing your health nutritionally and in other ways, leaving you with a weakened immune system.

> "The common varieties of tapeworm are acquired by human beings through eating raw or imperfectly cooked beef, pork, or sausage" (6)

The question is, why would any sane person want to cook and eat any meat product which contain tapeworms. Remember you will not be only eating cooked meat, but also cooked tapeworm which is still disturbing, why not make better choices?

> "We know that the flesh of animals is not necessary for anyone; that flesh foods are not our best sources of proteins and fats; that everything we get from flesh, except its content of animal waste, its diseased portions and the putrefactive poisons it contains, may be had in better and more usable conditions from many other foods, especially nuts." (7)

Yes, the obsession with meat is so great that better, healthier choices are overlooked. The plant kingdom has such a wide variety of healthy, nutritious, delicious foods, without the baggage which present day meat carries.

"We do not yet know the cause of many human diseases such as arthritis, collagen disease, the wasting muscle diseases, many of the chronic and disabling intestinal diseases (Crohn's disease, ulcerative, colitis, cilia disease, and fibrocystic disease of the pancreas), many of the crippling neurological diseases, and on and on. It is not a far-fetched idea that many of these diseases of unknown cause are related to animal diseases transmitted to man either by direct contact with the animal or by ingestion of the flesh, milk or eggs of the infected animal. (8)

The truth of the matter is, mass produced animal products are not generally 100% safe as can be seen by the known recalls, and outbreak of various health hazards. Then there are the silent dangers, the ones which take years to manifest themselves, which entail a lot of unnecessary pain and suffering.

"Raw and undercooked fish can harbor parasites that cause infection. Although the problem is not severe in North American waters, it does exist, says Terry Dick, Ph. D., Professor of Zoology of the University of Manitoba … Cold smoked salmon and other raw fish can also harbor parasites …"(9)

A problem being not severe is OK if you are not infected, but that doesn't give any comfort to an infected person. And the madness about this is some people do eat raw fish.

"Consuming infected meat or milk may result in a condition named campylobacter enteritis after the organism involved. Outbreaks occur particularly in schools or are contracted from pets, and are characterized by a slow onset of fever, nausea, muscular pains and abdominal pain, sometimes confused with appendicitis. This is followed by profuse, offensive and often bloodstained diarrhea the next day which may be so severe as to cause incontinence and may last for several weeks." (10)

This is another problem, which can be life threatening or even fatal. You get sick from eating infected meat or milk or even contracted from pets, then you are misdiagnosed, and treated for something else.And all this could have been easily avoided.

"The common tapeworms are of two varieties: beef and pork tapeworms, caused by eating of the raw or imperfectly cooked meats." (11)

There has been a deterioration in the quality of even beef as tapeworms are found in it, making it a health risk.I think, it is not just about imperfection in the cooking, but also imperfection in rearing these animals.Why, with all this modern science can there be some method to eliminate the tapeworms from infecting the beef?

"Washington - A new, sometimes fatal form of E. coli bacteria is now so prevalent in beef that it is no longer possible to guarantee the safety of hamburger, a panel of experts said yesterday.The panel of scientists, policy makers and meat industry representatives that yesterday urged cobalt-type radiation of most ground beef before it is marketed as a way to kill off the bacteria." (12)

Just what I said earlier, why can't all this hyped up science "prevent" rather than just try to kill off the bacteria?

"Viruses are anywhere from ten to one thousand times smaller than bacteria, and bacteria are microscopic, single celled animals ... (E. coli bacteria live by the millions in your intestines.)" (13)

I will comment on this, after reference 14.

"E. coli 0157:H7 acquired such startling capacities to sicken and kill by mutilating probably in the 1970 's – to contain two genes for manufacture of powerful toxins.Antibiotics are useless against the organism. The drugs kill the bacteria, but upon death the organisms release all their toxins, flooding the victim's body with deadly poison." (14)

Now, this is really scary, as the bacteria gets revenge, even after it dies. So the antibiotics are really useless, or rather deadly in this case.My reasoning is, the mad obsession of eating meat, even if it sickens you, has got to stop. The whole point is that beef with E. coli bacteria is neither safe, good or healthy to eat, and all this spring from the way the animals are reared.

You have to take control of your health, and say, this is where I stop this madness in my eating preferences.

"Chicken feed had poisonous arsenic (to speed growth), antibiotics, tranquilizers, anti infective agents, aspirin, stilbestrol, and pesticides. These chemical, poisonous drugs get into the chicken flesh and are eaten by the consumer.' (15)

More madness, how can chickens fed all those poisons, be ever safe to eat, even though the spices and seasoning make them look and smell good? Do you think there was any thought about the consumers health and well-being down the line or the health of the chicken?

"In Michigan and several other areas, diphyllobothrium latum the fish tapeworm, has been identified in man … The fish tapeworm normally lives in the subarctic and temperate regions. It is the largest tapeworm found in man. (16).

Even fish, once thought as a safe healthy alternative to beef and chicken are contaminated, and the tapeworm is transmitted to man, and it is also the largest.

Again, I cannot stress enough, God has created so much food in abundance for us which are not only safe, but delicious and nutritious, why can't we explore that field and make use of them, fruits, vegetables, nuts, seeds etc?

"There are more than one thousand eight hundred strains of salmonella bacteria, and most of them can cause food poisoning. But there are other culprits too. Staphylococcus aureus, Clostridium botulinum, and Clostridium perfringens are three of the most well known …Unfortunately, all … of these bacteria are everywhere. Most fish and poultry, for example, are contaminated by salmonella before they even get to your home.

So rather than trying to get rid of these bacteria – actually an impossible task - preventing their growth or killing them before they attack is the only way you can protect yourself ." (17)

The comment after reference 16 is applicable here

"Bees have only recently been recognized as a cause of disease in humans. The virus which causes acute bee paralysis has properties similar to those of pircorna viruses, the name given to a group of small RNA viruses which belong to the entro viruses and the rhino viruses.They cause intestinal and upper respiratory diseases respectively …Botulism from honey has been reported in infants under the age of six months." (18)

After reading all this information from disease sources, how can people still be indifferent.What people in general, including Muslims have to understand, it's not just about eating, as in the Qur'an, Allah says over and over, "eat of the good things", so even plants are messed up by genetic engineering and do you think when bees use pollen from those plants' flowers that the results will be good?

There was great concern about bees dying, in an article I read in a newspaper, also in a magazine, as bees play important roles in our existence.

So as we have seen, just eating any chicken, cow, fish turkey etc, which were loaded with poisonous toxins, are not healthy choices, and that goes for all genetically modified fruits, vegetables and plants.

"Newborn infants may contact listeriosis, disease that causes fever during pregnancy, but ' usually undiagnosed. The baby gets the germ during passage through the birth canal or is infected from environmental sources. Cows, goats, sheep, hogs poultry (especially turkeys), fish, crabs, and rabbits are known reservoirs of the disease." (19)

Look at the long list, and this still will not deter some people from eating them.And the holiday indoctrination of eating turkey on thanksgiving day continues, and in this instance, the turkey is the main culprit. Look at the many advertisements on TV, the Newspapers, magazines, books etc., with so many pictures of all those species, and nothing is given as a warning.

When drugs are advertised as a cure(?) for anything, they list a whole lot of side effects, what a cure. The same standard should be made for all those beef, mutton, pork, chicken, turkey, crab, lobster and fish, there should be a list of dangers that may accompany eating them.

"Many farm by-products are salvaged for use as animal feeds. Since these are spent materials, much of their original nutritional value is lost. The Farmers' Weekly (England) reported: "a group of housed pregnant sheep on a special food which has dried poultry manure as its Protein base" The ewes were a bit put off by the taste, but this has been overcome by adding molasses and chicory." (20)

More mad science, is this how God intended these animals to be treated? When they eat filth, and you eat them, do you expect to be healthy?

"Let us review this point in the context of cancer. For years, the United States Food and Drug Administration permitted the chicken and cattle in industries to speed the marketing of their meat by administering to the fowl and animals quantities of stilbestrol, a synthetic form of female hormone.

Certain medical men and certain of us in public health education were convinced that stilbestrol is capable of causing cancer. It has long been known that male chemists occupied in synthesizing this hormone are apt to develop cancer of the breast, an extremely rare occurrence in men. The cancer is probably caused by exposure to the stilbestrol dust in the laboratory … Then under public pressure, the Food and Drug Administration reversed its stand. It announced that the cancer causing action of the hormone made its use in the chicken industry unsafe, though the ruling still allowed the beef producer to employ the substance." (21)

What thought is given to the effect all this, will have on the consumer, is it just the dollars that matter?

"In an effort to salvage inedible tallow and grease, the USDA is developing methods of adding them to livestock feed. Tasteless food grade plastic has been made into artificial roughage pellets for cattle on high concentrate or all-grain rations. Ground-up newspapers, mixed with molasses, have been fed to cattle at Pennsylvania State University. Feathers have also been used as a supplement in animal food at the College of Agriculture at Missouri …" (22)

Imagine feeding vegetarian animals with processed tallow, then to add insult to injury, plastic and newspapers being added. You have a brain in your head, use it before it's gone, how can all that nonsense be beneficial to those animals health and in extension by eating them, yours?

"We are all aware, from news stories that certain food additives, including sprays and processing materials, have been shown to be cancer-causing. Some of these chemicals produce, among other things, an oxygen deficiency in the cells, and it has been established that a cellular oxygen deficiency will help produce cancer." (23)

This can give you a hint why cancer is on the rise, and after so many years and billions of dollars, they can't find a cure.If you are using your brain you can easily see "the cure".If you can't see "the cure", my question to you, why are you still consuming food products that are cancerous?

The Almighty Creator has put in everyone of us the cure for all diseases "OUR IMMUNE SYSTEMS" and remember that it must be nourished properly to be able to function properly.

> "As a result, the basic physiology of the animal has been altered. For example, young beef animals, twelve to eighteen months old. may be confined to feedlots and encouraged to overeat fattening foods. Drugs may also be given that change the metabolism and increase fat artificially. This fat is hard, white and almost totally saturated. Over the years slaughterhouses workers have noted the differences in the appearance of the fat, flesh, and organs of these animals." (24)

I have been saying this for years on end, that the basic physiology of animals have been altered, by the garbage they are being fed, and worse by genetic engineering.Even some plants have had their natural genetic make-up messed up by genetic engineering.All that mad science are producing and will continue to produce, disease, suffering, disablement and painful deaths in humans who consume those products.

> "Frozen fish is good food, too, though its origin in the sea does not protect you, as some people have supposed, against the insecticides to which cattle have been exposed. Sprays are used in the wholesale fish market, as well as on the farm." (25)

And also from smaller fish which eat waste from prescription drugs, and other contaminants in the water, then bigger fish eat them, and so up the food chain, then humans eat them.

"Antibiotics added to animal feed, make young calves grow at a faster rate. This shortens the growing period and makes them ready for market sooner. Many antibiotics, used for this purpose, now supplement animal feed. In as such many bacteria have become resistant to the older antibiotics, newer and stronger ones are added to an ever-growing growing list." (26)

Do they not think that speeding up the growth of those animals artificially will have disastrous effects, long term, in them and the consumers?

"I have seen and heard first hand what goes on in the poultry rearing. I saw dead chickens, trampled by other chickens, and their flesh looked blue. The man in charge of rearing them, told me that it was unsafe to eat them before a certain time period, which allowed the drugs to leave their system. Then the color of the flesh returned to normal. But what guarantees do we have?

Remember, too, all the warnings about "Salmonella" in eggs. Must we take these chances with our well being when there is a safe alternative? Even the seas, lakes, and rivers, which at one point in time were considered good sources of healthy food, are risky. Fish now are very hazardous to eat, contaminated somewhere along the line by pesticides, industrial chemicals, parasites, natural toxins, toxic metals, microorganisms, etc.Damage to the human system from eating contaminated fish ranges from cancer, damage to the human nerve cells, kidney damage, hearing problems, damage to your mental development, visual problems, etc" (27)

A final word, is it worth the risk considering the dangers involved, what is this mad obsession with animal products consumption at all costs.Many diseases and ailments can be cured, just by changing your diet, why take in all these poisonous toxins and mess up your metabolism and other bodily functions, why?

References

1. Chicago Sun-Times Thursday July 25, 1996 pages 12, 13

2. The Animal Connection by Agatha Thrash MD and Calvin Thrash M. D. page 3

3. Understanding Disease - A Health Practitioners Handbook by John Ball page 46

4. African Holistic Health by Llaila O. Afrika page 128

5. Fighting Disease by Ellen Michaud, Alice Feinsein and The Editors of Prevention Magazine page 221

6. The Family Physician by Dr. Herman Pomenanz and Dr. Irvin S. Koll page 294

7. Superior Nutrition by H. M. Shelton page 71

8. The Animal Connection by Agatha Thrash MD and Calvin Thrash M. D. page 2

9. Fighting Disease by Ellen Michaud, Alice Feinstein and The Editors of Prevention Magazine page 225

10. Understanding Disease - A Health Practitioners Handbook by John Ball page 40

11. The Family Physician by Dr. Herman Pomeranz and Dr. Irvin S. Koll page 296

12. New York Newsday - Thursday July 14, 1994

13. Fighting Disease by Ellen Michaud, Alice Feinstein and The Editors of Prevention Magazine page 309

14. New York Newsday - Thursday July 14, 1994 from article FDA Burgers Can Be Risky. pages A4 to A5

15. African Holistic Health by Llaila O. Afrika page 129

16. The Animal Connection by Agatha Thrash M.D and Calvin Thrash M. D. page 8

17. Fighting Disease by Ellen Michaud, Alice Feinstein and The Editors of Prevention Magazine page 157

18. The Animal Connection by Agatha Thrash M.D and Calvin Thrash M. D. page 8

19. The Animal Connection by Agatha Thrash M.D and Calvin Thrash M. D. page 20

20. Consumer Beware by Beatrice Trum Hunter page 113

21. Food Facts and Fallacies by Carlton Fredericks, Ph. D. and Herbert Bailey page 82

22. Consumer Beware by Beatrice Trum Hunter page 113

23. Food Facts and Fallacies by Carlton Fredericks, Ph. D. and Herbert Bailey page 82

24. Consumer Beware by Beatrice Trum Hunter page 112

25. Food Facts and Fallacies by Carlton Fredericks, Ph. D. and Herbert Bailey page 286

26. A Taste of Mama Nature - A Handbook for Vegans and Vegetarians with Recipes and Exercise Plan by Abolade Nkosi Tayo page 86

CHAPTER 9

DISEASES PASSED ON FROM ANIMALS (PETS) TO HUMANS

Another vehicle for diseases passed on to humans by animals and often overlooked and played down, are by way of pets. You can see children hugging dogs, cats, rabbits, playing with white mice and even kissing these animals, and they assume that these practices are harmless, think again, as what you will read is going to jolt you.

"Generally speaking, cats are more likely than dogs to spread disease to children and household members. Furthermore, cats more than other pets spread disease to dogs and other companion animals. Cats are a threat to humans by their many diseases, including rabies.Cat bites, scratches, or fleas from cats may transmit several kinds of infection." (1)

"Cats (toxoplasmosis) and even parrots (psittacosis) are examples of the variety of possible vectors. It is in fact a protozoan and spreads to humans from cats, in the intestines of which it reproduces itself. The cat excretes the cysts and these are spread either direct to humans through cat litter trays and gardens, or else ingested by other animals such as goats, sheep and pigs." (2)

"Almost anyone who owns a pet cat and tends kitty's Litter box comes in contact with yet another protozoan – the microscopic creature that causes toxoplasmosis.

The real danger with toxoplasmosis is to pregnant women. If the parasite infects a woman while she is pregnant, the infection can kill her unborn child or cause blindness and other birth defects."Pregnant women should avoid cats as much as possible," advises Dr. Duncan."(3)

I admit that some animals bring comfort to some people, but they also can bring some other very unpleasant things, as can be seen from references 1, 2, 3.

They range from infections, spreading diseases to children and adults, also dangers to pregnant women, as their unborn children can have birth defects or even die.

Sometimes or rather most of the times people get sick, in homes with animals, usually they are overlooked as the source of the sickness.For the simple reason, they assume that their pets are clean and healthy.

"A very similar type of ringworm, Tinea capitis, can be caught from animals like dogs and cats and affects mainly the scalp. An inflamed and itchy area develops and the hair may be lost in a manner similar to alopecia from which it must be differentiated." (4)

The ringworm caught from animals like dogs and cats could be all over any house they live in.I have seen dogs which run free outdoors after they defecate, they squat down and drag their butts on the grass, I saw cats doing the same thing.

But what about cats and dogs in the house how do they clean up after their numbers, well, the carpet or the couch are good places, and cats who like to climb, it could be on your bed or some higher place, like your kitchen counter etc.

"Cat Bite. The bite of any animal may transmit rabies to the victim
...

The cat's mouth incidentally, contains germs that are more dangerous
to human beings than the germs found in a dog's mouth ...Dog
Bite. The prevention of hydrophobia is extremely important" (5)

In the cat's mouth ,there are more dangerous germs to humans than those
in a dog's mouth:yet still, I have seen children and adults kissing cats in
their mouths, and they do it without a concern for their health and well-
being.

Psittacosis, a pulmonary disease with fever, shortness of breath,
cough and other respiratory tract symptoms can be contracted from
birds. The mortality rate is five to ten per cent. Patients often do
not suspect that they have caught a disease from birds. Pet hamsters
have been the source of an outbreak of lyphocytic choriomeningitis,
a disease characteristically producing a fever, headache and severe
muscle aches." (6)

A few years ago, in New York, I visited a home and I saw a small child
(about two years old) hugging a cat in bed, and he (the child) had a runny
nose.

I told his mother, that if she puts the cat outside the apartment, and keep
the child away from it, his runny nose would stop. She reluctantly followed
my advice, and as I told her, his runny nose stopped.

I have seen cats climb all over peoples' furniture, dining tables, stoves and
all imaginable places.

In 2014, I saw a newspaper picture, spread out on a whole page tabloid
size, about a woman who owns a restaurant.The picture was taken in her
kitchen, where she was preparing some food, what was really disturbing is
that she sat on a chair preparing food, on the dining table nearly, was this
big dog, looking down, and right next to her was another dog.

Now you tell me, if this is not a case of really careless, unhealthy food preparation.I don't eat out, so I won't be going to her Restaurant.Some people think it's OK to have their dogs, and cats running around in their kitchen, when preparing food.

I have seen people play with their pets, then go right on to hold a sandwich or some other food item, without washing their hands, this is really sickening.Then there is a double whammy, you take the animal out of their natural environment (outdoors), and bring them into your home, feeding them a lot of processed foods. They end up with the same diseases plaguing mankind, who eat processed foods (arthritis, diabetes, hemorrhoids etc), and they in turn give you their diseases, what a horrible exchange.

Don't get me wrong, I love animals, this is why I don't approve of the way some farm animals are treated.I know that some animals perform good services, I know all this, but the craze of just wanting animals in your house, is not a healthy choice, weigh the matter carefully, especially when children and pregnant women are involved.

References

1. The Animal Connection by Agatha Thrash MD and Calvin Thrash M. D. page 17

2. Understanding Disease - A Health Practitioners Handbook by John Ball pages 42, 43

3. Fighting Disease by Ellen Michaud, Alice Feinstein and The Editors of Prevention Magazine page 226

4. Understanding Disease - A Health Practitioners Handbook by John Ball page 56

5. The Family Physician by Dr. Herman Pomeranz and Dr. Irvin S. Koll page 518

6. The Animal Connection by Agatha Thrash MD and Calvin Thrash M. D. page 19

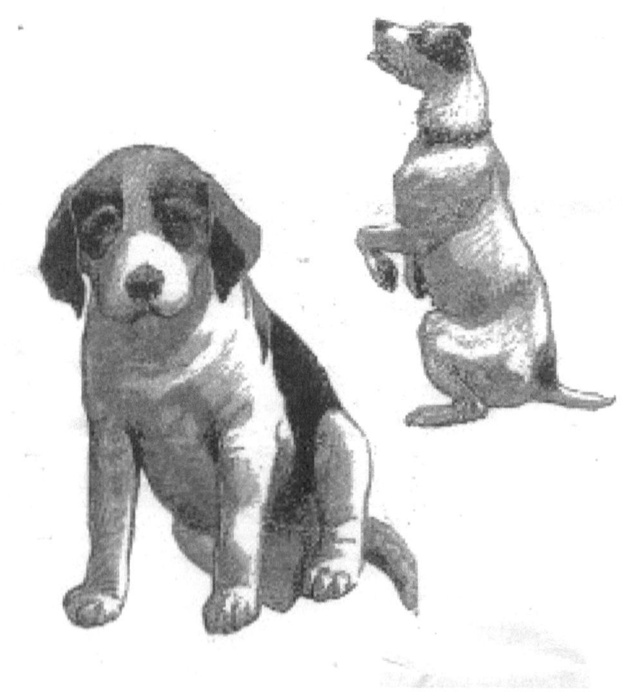

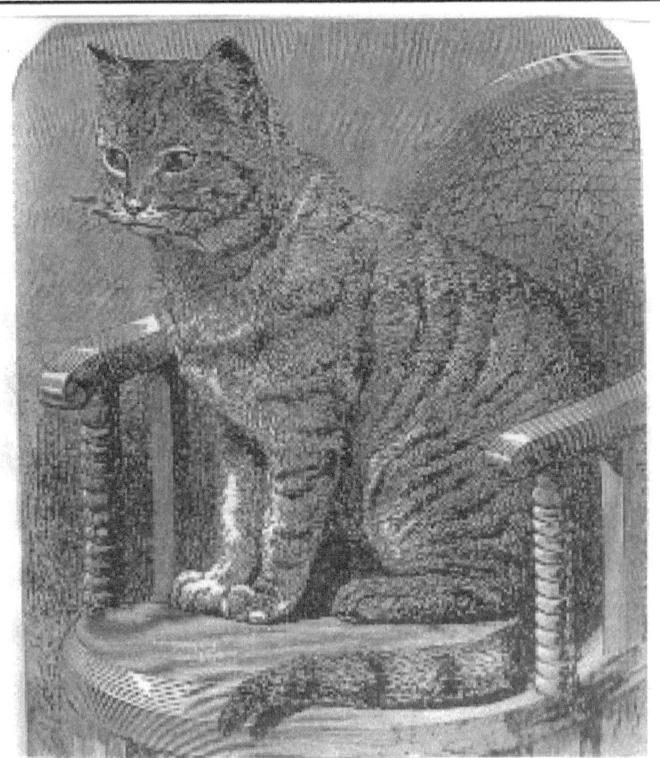

AFTERWORD

After all the products listed as containing pork by products, here are some guidelines to using pork free products.

Use only vegetable based soap for taking a shower, or those which state no animal products. Try to purchase your fruits, apples, pears from organic producers or wash questionable ones under warm water or submerge them in hot water, wash with Liquid Black soap diluted in water ,then peel before eating.

Do not buy pigskin leather bags etc, use "vegetable based and herbal toothpaste."

Do not use genetically modified produce, check the PLU #.

You must use your brain, why kill the bacteria, virus and all the other contaminants which go with the product, your best choice is to avoid them.

It is better and wiser to eat fresh organic plant produce,or non-gmo conventional grown produce , rather than go through the myriad of so-called measures in those questionable food items discussed in this book.

APPRECIATION

All Praises and Thanks be to Allah the One Who has permitted me to write this book and the One Who made me intelligent.

I thank my mother (now deceased) for the great effort she made in educating me, with the little resources at her disposal, may Allah have mercy on her.

I thank my stepmother (Carmen) my father's wife(recently deceased). She was very kind to me and always encouraged me in all my projects. May Allah have mercy on her.

I thank my step father (Bertie Antoine-now deceased) who I grew up with, who read a lot, and I gained much from him, may Allah have mercy on him.

I thank my father (now deceased) who read a lot and this in some way inspired me to read also, may Allah have mercy on him.

I thank my daughter Dara who typesetted and edited the original edition of this book, may Allah bless and guide her.

I thank Bernard Borde whom I consider as my brother. He was kind to me, listened to my plans, supported me and wished me well. May Allah bless and guide him.

I thank Yoel who stretched out his hand to me when I needed help. May Allah bless and guide him.

I thank Edgar Henry who as a professional always found time to exchange notes and ideas with me even though he was busy. May Allah bless and guide him.

I thank Rafi who I love as a son, he is "MY TRUE SON",who encouraged me to concentrate on publishing and marketing my books.Who unselfishly stretched out his hand to help me in numerous ways and many times. May Allah guide, bless, protect and give him success in this life and more in the Hereafter

I thank my daughter Ayodele who stretched out her hand to me, not only to help me, but to be close to me, to make sure I am taken care of. May Allah guide, bless, protect and give her success in this life and more in the Hereafter.

I thank Asaru, who we fondly call Ru for all the help, encouragement, effort and the many constructive conversations we have had, he is an excellent student. He has learnt a lot from me, hopefully he will continue in his never ending quest for knowledge, and carry on a great part of my work when I am gone. May Allah guide him on His Right path and make it easy for him on his journey.

I thank Wayne Joseph (Junior) who we fondly call Trini for all the help, assistance and encouragement he has given me and my family.I count him as a son, may Allah guide him to his truth.

I thank Angela Rosario who I fondly call Angie, who has helped me in so many ways, who is the one most responsible for me being able to use the computer. She patiently spent time teaching me how to navigate the system.

She spent time in typing some of my books, she sat me down, and let me know that I was important, that the work I was doing at a facility where she was my Supervisor,was important as when you look all around you can see what I have done. She encouraged me in my aspirations, she was always concerned about my welfare, I thank you Angie and may Allah reward you.

I thank Dr. Altaf who addresses me, as Uncle, I love him as if he was my biological nephew. He was always happy to see me, and made time to speak to me. Over the years he has helped me, my family and was always concerned about my welfare and also my family's. May Allah bless him, guide him ,richly reward him in this life and more in the Hereafter.

I thank all those who have helped me over the years Imam Khalifah, Imam Ibrahim, Gamali, Dawud, Bill, Bentley (Jawanza) ,Ajamu,and many others who I have not mentioned by name, may Allah reward you all and make your paths easy.

I thank Janet Good, the one who means so much to me. The one who shares my dreams. The one who stood by me and supported me,encouraged me,loved me,and Insha Allah,the one who would share in my success.

RECOMMENDED READING

The Animal Connection by Agatha Thrash, MD and Calvin Thrash, MD

The Hog – Should It Be Used As Food? By C. Leonard Vories

What The Holy Qur'an, Bible and Medical Say About Pork By Din Rana

African Holistic Health By Llaila O Afrika

How Not To Eat Pork By Shahrazad Ali

Disturbing Consequences By Abolade Nkosi Tayo

Science Gone Mad By Abolade Nkosi Tayo

Superior Nutrition By H.M. Shelton

Simple Nutrition By Abolade Nkosi Tayo

There is a Cure By Abolade Nkosi Tayo

Healthy Blender Recipes By Abolade Nkosi Tayo

Juicing For Good Health By Abolade Nkosi Tayo

BOOKS BY ABOLADE NKOSI TAYO

- ❖ There Is A Cure

- ❖ Disturbing Consequences

- ❖ Juicing for Good Health

- ❖ Healthy Blender Recipes

- ❖ Pork Eating The Great Risk To Human Health

- ❖ Simple Nutrition

- ❖ Soups – The Best Cooked Food

- ❖ Original Nutrition

- ❖ Science Gone Mad

- ❖ Afrika! The True Origin Of Karate And All Martial Arts

- ❖ Some Interesting Facts About Asa Kiniun (Simba Ryu) Afrikan Martial Arts

- ❖ Caribbean Folk Tales

- ❖ Ghosts, Jinn Or Natural Phenomena-Which?

- ❖ Reincarnation or Memory Transfer-Which?

- ❖ Is the Bible A Reliable Guide to Spiritual Truth?

- ❖ Jehovah Is Not The Name Of The Almighty Creator

- ❖ Who Founded Christianity – Paul or Jesus?

- ❖ The Crucifixion and Resurrection of Jesus Christ – Historical Fact Or Religious Fiction?

❖ The Paganism In Some Christian Churches

❖ China 2030 – The Rise Of The Last Superpower. Science-fiction.

To place an order go to

To order books go to http://lulu.com/spotlight/nkosi2020

❖ The Paganism In Some Christian Churches

❖ China 2030 – The Rise Of The Last Superpower. Science-fiction.

To place an order go to

To order books go to http://lulu.com/spotlight/nkosi2020

- Trichinosis causes fever, muscle aches and swelling around the eyes.

- The ordinary tapeworm is from twenty to fifty feet long.

- Our present hog crop may provide us with over 60,000,000 trichinae infested meals.

- Hot dogs are a potential source of a type of organism causing sporotrichinosis, a skin disease characterized by a string of molecules developing upward along the path of the lymphatic.

- Hookworms are spread to man by the consumption of pork.

- The pigs were actually used for two purposes, to clean up the mess, and then to be sold as pork.

- After reading some of the diseases spread to man by eating pork, I ask the following questions:

  * Is it ethical to be arrogant about the health of people by saying "What will we do with all these diseased dead hogs?"

  * What about "Mad-cow disease would it affect you?

  * What about religious people who eat meat, but don't eat hog? Is it fair to them?

  * The diseases spread to humans by animals

Published and distributed by Abolade Nkosi Tayo